MELANOMA

HEALTHY APPROACH FOR TREATING MELANOMA

DR. A. RAMOS

Contents

Introduction

Melanoma is a kind of skin cancer that arises from melanocytes, which are cells that create color. These cells create melanin, the pigment that gives skin, hair, and eyes their color. Melanoma is known to have the potential to grow into an aggressive tumor and spread to other parts of the body.

Crucial Information about Melanoma

Melanoma is caused by melanocytes, which are primarily found in the skin but are also present in the eyes, mucous membranes, and other parts of the body.

Dangerous Components

Sun Exposure: Extended or severe exposure to ultraviolet (UV) light from the sun or tanning beds can be quite dangerous.

Fair Skin: People with light skin tones, light hair, and light-colored eyes are generally more susceptible.

Family History: The risk is increased if there is a history of melanoma in the family or if the condition runs in the family.

ABCDE Rule of Detection:

The two halves of the mole are not equal, or asymmetric.

Border irregularity: The borders of the mole have an uneven or notch-shaped form.

Color: The mole's internal pigments may vary in hue.

Diameter: Melanomas often have a diameter larger than the tip of a pencil.

Evolution: Changes in size, shape, color, or altitude throughout time.

Types of Melanoma:

The most common type, called superficial spreading melanoma, is often characterized by irregularly shaped spots.

Nodular Melanoma: This type of cancer typically grows faster and appears higher.

Lentigo Maligna Melanoma: Usually affecting the elderly, this ailment manifests itself on areas that have been exposed to sunlight on a regular basis.

Acral lentiginous melanoma is a common condition that is generally found on the palms, soles, or under the nails; it is not usually associated with sun exposure.

Location:

Melanoma staging takes into account the tumor's thickness, whether it has spread to nearby lymph nodes, and whether it has spread to other organs.

Counseling:

Treatment options include immunotherapy, targeted therapy, radiation therapy, chemotherapy, and surgical excision.

The best likelihood of healing is achieved with surgical removal and early discovery.

Avoidance

Avoiding excessive sun exposure, using sunscreen, dressing in protective clothing, and regularly monitoring your skin are all part of prevention.

Individuals who are particularly vulnerable such as those with fair skin tones or a family history of the condition may need to be watched closely.

Melanoma is a severe kind of skin cancer that requires immediate medical attention. Regular skin checks and sun protection are crucial for people who are at risk because early detection and treatment significantly enhance results.

CHAPTER ONE

Definition of melanoma

Melanocytes, or color-producing cells, are the source of melanoma, a type of skin cancer. These cells create melanin, the pigment that gives skin, hair, and eyes their color. A malignant tumor called melanoma can develop in the skin or, less commonly, in other organs containing melanocytes, such as the eyes or mucous membranes. The malignant alteration of melanocytes is the cause of this.

Because melanoma tends to spread aggressively to other parts of the body, early diagnosis and treatment are critical to a favorable outcome. It often presents as changes in the appearance existing moles or as the appearance of new pigmented skin lesions.

Many risk factors, including sun exposure, pale skin, family history, and specific genetic characteristics, can contribute to the development of melanoma. The ABCDE rule, which stands for Asymmetry, Border irregularity, Color variations, Diameter greater than a pencil eraser, and Evolution or changes over time, is a helpful tool for recognizing potential signs of melanoma.

The features that establish the stage of melanoma include the tumor's thickness, whether it has spread to nearby lymph nodes, and whether it has spread to other organs. Treatment options for melanoma may include immunotherapy, targeted therapy, chemotherapy, and radiation therapy, depending on its stage and characteristics.

Prevention strategies include sun protection practices like applying sunscreen, donning protective clothing, and frequently inspecting one's skin. Early diagnosis and therapy are critical to improving prognosis for melanoma patients.

It is essential to comprehend melanoma and diagnose it early.

Understanding and detecting melanoma at an early stage is critical for several reasons:

1. Increased Success Rates

Early recognition significantly increases the chances of recovery. Surgery is often a very successful treatment when melanoma is detected early and is contained.

2. Keeping Metastasis at Bay:

Melanoma has the potential to metastasize, or spread, to other bodily areas. The condition can be prevented from advancing to a more advanced and difficult stage that calls for more intensive medical care by receiving early diagnosis and treatment.

3. Procedure for Surgery:

In its early stages, surgical excision alone is often sufficient to treat melanoma. When the only condition found is skin cancer, surgical removal of the tumor is a less invasive and simpler procedure.

4. Decreasing the Severity of Care:

Early-stage melanomas may respond better to less aggressive treatment than those with more advanced stages. The individual might have a better quality of life and have fewer side effects as a result.

5. Increased Survival Rates:

Greater survival rates are linked to early identification of melanoma. Early intervention makes treatment more successful overall and improves overall results.

6. Reduced Medical Costs:

Early detection can lead to simpler and less expensive treatment solutions. The cost of treating advanced-stage melanoma and its aftereffects is high.

7. Patient Empowerment:

Individuals who receive early detection are more capable of taking care of their own health. Regular skin inspections and monitoring of changes in pigmented lesions or moles provide proactive health management.

8. Quality of Life:

Early treatment may mitigate the detrimental consequences of the condition on an individual's physical and emotional well-being by maintaining the skin's typical function and look.

9. Preventive measures:

By identifying those who are more prone to acquire melanoma, tailored preventative measures, such as increased sun protection and regular skin tests, can be put into place.

10. Effect on Learning:

Recognizing the importance of prompt detection raises awareness of skin cancer risks and encourages adoption of sun safety behaviors. Education is the main factor in melanoma prevention.

11. Investigations and Clinical Trials:

Early detection makes it easier to participate in clinical trials and research studies, which is why advancements in melanoma therapy and management can be linked to it.

Early melanoma detection is critical to successfully managing skin cancer. Regular skin inspections, being aware of changes in moles or skin lesions, and prompt medical intervention can all help people who are at risk of developing melanoma or who have already been diagnosed with the disease to achieve better outcomes and general well-being.

Understanding Melanoma

Learning about melanoma include becoming familiar with its characteristics, risk factors, detection techniques, and accessible therapies. Here's a thorough summary:

1. Features of melanoma include:

Melanoma originates from melanocytes, which are the cells that produce color in the skin.

Aggression: The ability of melanoma to spread aggressively to other body parts is widely known.

There are several different types of melanoma, including nodule, lentigo maligna, acral lentiginous, and superficial spreading melanoma.

2. Dangerous Components

Sun Exposure: Prolonged or strong exposure to ultraviolet (UV) radiation, especially from the sun, is one of the key risk factors.

Fair Skin: Victims are more likely to have fair skin, light hair, and light-colored eyes.

If melanoma runs in the family, the risk is higher.

Genetic Factors: Individuals with particular genetic mutations may be more prone to melanoma.

3. Locating and Identifying:

According to the ABCDE Rule, asymmetry, uneven borders, color changes, diameter more than a pencil eraser, and evolution or changes over time are all significant signs of potential melanoma.

Skin Exams: Both routine self-examinations and professional skin examinations are crucial for early detection.

Biopsy: Usually performed to confirm the diagnosis, a biopsy involves removing a sample of the suspicious skin lesion for investigation.

4. Location:

TNM System: Factors such as tumor thickness, lymph node involvement, and distant metastases are considered for staging melanoma.

5. Treatment Options:

Surgical Excision: When melanomas are still in their early stages, excision of the tumor is a popular treatment.

CHAPTER TWO

The purpose of sentinel lymph node biopsies is to determine whether nearby lymph nodes have been affected by cancer.

Immunotherapy: Medication used in immunotherapy helps the immune system identify and get rid of melanoma cells.

Medication that specifically targets certain biochemical pathways connected to the advancement of melanoma is known as targeted treatment.

Chemotherapy: While less common for melanoma, conventional chemotherapy can be used under certain conditions.

6. Avoidance

Sun Protection: Applying sunscreen, finding shade, and donning protective gear all help reduce the chance of developing melanoma.

Regular Skin Checks: Early detection is crucial, especially in individuals with risk factors, and can only be achieved by professional skin checks and self-examinations.

7. Adaptability and Follow-Up:

Survivorship Plans: Patients are provided with plans that outline monitoring and aftercare after treatment.

Psychosocial Support: Maintaining one's emotional and mental well-being is crucial to melanoma survival.

8. Present-day Studies:

Advances: Present research endeavors explore new avenues for treatment, early identification methods, and prophylactic actions for melanoma.

Understanding melanoma requires a multimodal approach that takes into account risk factors, early detection methods, available therapies, and ongoing research projects. Thanks to this comprehensive understanding, people can now take proactive steps for prevention, early intervention, and overall skin health.

Contributors to Hazards

Skin cancer that is more likely to develop if specific risk factors are satisfied is called melanoma. Individuals who are aware of these risk factors are more likely to identify issues early on and take action to avoid problems from developing. Some of the main risk factors for melanoma are as follows:

1. Sunlight Absorption:

Prolonged Exposure to High UV Radiation: UV radiation, mostly from the sun, is quite dangerous.

Sunburns: Having a history of severe sunburns increases your risk, particularly if they happened while you were a baby or teenager.

2. Skin Type and Pigmentation:

Fair complexion: Individuals with fair complexion, light-colored eyes, and fair hair are more susceptible.

Diminished Pigmentation: Lower melanin levels result in a lessened skin's natural defense against UV exposure.

3. Individual and Family History:

Family History: Having a parent, sibling, or child who is a first-degree relative and has a history of melanoma increases your risk.

Personal History: If a person has a history of melanoma or other skin cancers, their risk is elevated.

4. Genetic Components:

Genetic Mutations: Certain genetic mutations, such as those in the CDKN2A gene, are associated with an increased risk of melanoma.

Genetic Syndromes: Individuals with certain syndromes, such as familial atypical multiple mole melanoma (FAMMM), may be at an increased risk of developing melanoma.

5. Sunburns and the use of tanning beds:

Severe Sunburns: Frequent incidence of severe sunburns, especially those that blister, increases the risk.

Tanning Beds: Using tanning beds exposes users to ultraviolet radiation, which increases the risk of melanoma.

6. Age and Gender:

Age: Although melanoma can occur at any age, as people age, their risk increases. Senior citizens are more likely to experience it.

Gender: In younger people, melanoma is slightly more common in women, but in elderly people, it is more common in men.

7. Diminished Immune Reaction:

Immunosuppression: Individuals with weakened immune systems, such as recipients of organ transplants or those suffering from particular diseases, are more susceptible.

8. Typical and Atypical Moles:

Many Moles: Having a large number of moles (nevi) on one's skin is associated with an increased risk.

Dysplastic Nevi (Atypical Moles): The risk may be higher if you have dysplastic nevi or atypical moles.

9. Workplace Exposures:

Occupational Hazards: Certain occupational exposures to carcinogens, such as coal tar or particular chemicals, may raise the risk.

10. Location of Geographic Origin:

High UV Index: Living in regions with high UV radiation levels, especially those nearer the equator, increases your risk.

People can adopt sun-safe behaviors, such as wearing protective clothing, frequently applying sunscreen, and closely monitoring their skin, by being aware of these risk factors. A family history of melanoma or other risk factors may make more frequent skin inspections and close monitoring by medical professionals beneficial for the affected individual. For individuals who are susceptible to melanoma, timely detection is crucial for better results.

Skin malignancies, including melanoma, can present with a variety of signs and symptoms. To obtain prompt medical attention and take appropriate action, it is imperative to recognize these early warning signs. Important signs and symptoms of melanoma include the following:

1. Changes in Moles (ABCDE Rule):

The two halves of the mole are not equal, or asymmetric.

Border irregularity: The borders of the mole are fuzzy, jagged, or marked with notch marks.

Variations in Color: The mole may show various shades of brown, black, red, or white.

Diameter: Melanomas often have a diameter of at least six mm, which is larger than the eraser on a pencil.

Evolution or Changes Over Time: It's critical to monitor any alterations to form, elevation, size, color, or other characteristics.

2. unusual or novel moles:

appearance of a mole that has just been found, especially beyond the age of 25, or the development of a mole that starts to stand out from the other moles that are already there.

3. Itching or Sensation:

Itching, pain, or sensitivity in a mole or on the skin's surface.

4. Alterations in Skin Texture:

changes, including roughening or scaling, to the texture of the skin around the mole.

5. Leaking or Streaming:

Any mole or skin lesion that bleeds or leaks fluid without obvious cause needs to be examined.

6. Dark Marks Undernails or on Palms and Soles:

the appearance of black streaks or lines on the foot's palms, soles, or beneath the nails.

7. Swelling, Redness, or Inflammation:

the development of inflammation, edema, or redness on the skin near a mole.

8. Satellite-Related Damage:

Lesions are little black spots that appear on the edges of preexisting moles.

9. Changes in Vision (Ocular Melanoma):

Symptoms of ocular melanoma may include changes in vision, seeing black patches, or experiencing visual impairment.

10. Bigger Lymph Nodes:

swelling or expansion of the surrounding lymph nodes, especially in the absence of pain.

It's important to keep in mind that melanoma can appear anywhere on the skin, including areas that are shielded from the sun. Moreover, melanoma can develop in the eyes or mucous membranes, like those in the mouth, genitalia, or anus.

Self-examination of the skin on a frequent basis, using the ABCDE rule, and seeking medical attention for any concerning changes are necessary for early detection. Risk factors include things like a personal history of skin cancer or a family history of melanoma. Dermatologists may find that patients with these disorders benefit from more regular skin exams and professional assessments. Prompt care and early detection are critical for improving the prognosis of melanoma patients.

Melanoma is diagnosed by a combination of imaging examinations, clinical examination, and most importantly a biopsy to confirm the presence of malignant cells. The following are crucial steps in the diagnosis of melanoma:

1. Clinical Evaluation:

Dermatological Examination: A dermatologist or other healthcare provider examines the skin and moles using a dermatoscope, a portable instrument that allows for a deeper examination.

A healthcare expert evaluates moles and skin lesions using the ABCDE criteria (Asymmetry, Border irregularity, Color variations, Diameter more than a pencil eraser, and Evolution or changes over time).

2. autopsy

Excisional Biopsy: The entire suspicious lesion or mole is excised, along with a margin of healthy skin. This is often the suggested course of action for small lesions.

Incisional Biopsy: A portion of the suspicious area is excised in order to evaluate it. This can be required if the lesion is large or in a delicate area.

3. Histopathological Examination:

Laboratory Analysis: The excised tissue is sent to a pathology laboratory for microscopic examination.

Determination of Cancer Kind and Stage: The pathologist not only determines the type of melanoma and whether the cells are malignant, but also provides information on the tumor's thickness and whether it has spread to other tissues.

4. Imaging Studies:

Sentinel Lymph Node Biopsy: When melanoma is suspected of having spread, a sentinel lymph node biopsy may be performed to determine whether cancer cells are present in the surrounding lymph nodes.

Imaging Tests: If there are signs that the disease is spreading, imaging tests such as CT, MRI, or

PET scans may be performed to assess the extent of metastasis to other organs.

5. Location:

TNM Staging System: When staging melanoma, factors such as tumor thickness, lymph node involvement, and the presence of distant metastases are taken into consideration.

6. Genetic Analysis:

BRAF Mutation Testing: In order to determine the most effective course of targeted therapy, genetic testing is occasionally performed to identify specific mutations, including BRAF mutations.

7. ocular melanoma detection by ocular examination

Ophthalmic Examination: In situations of ocular melanoma, an ophthalmologist examines the eye using particular techniques.

8. Multidisciplinary Teamwork Method:

Team Consultation: A multidisciplinary team comprising dermatologists, pathologists, oncologists, and other specialists collaborates to determine the optimal course of action.

Accurate staging and timely diagnosis are essential for developing a successful treatment plan. When melanoma is positively detected, doctors can tailor treatment plans to the particular characteristics of the cancer, improving the likelihood of successful outcomes. Individuals should get in touch with a doctor as soon as they discover changes in their skin or suspicious moles so that they can have a thorough examination and, if necessary, a biopsy.

Phase and Prospects

Determining the disease's course and guiding treatment decisions require accurate melanoma staging. The prognosis, or anticipated course of events, is influenced by the stage of melanoma at diagnosis. Staging is typically accomplished using the TNM technique, which considers the characteristics of the primary tumor (T), the involvement of nearby lymph nodes (N), and the presence of distant metastases (M). The following is a summary of melanoma stages and prognosis:

1. In Situ Melanoma, Stage 0:

Description: Malignant cells are only found in the epidermis, the skin's outermost layer.

It has an excellent prognosis. The malignancy has a good prognosis and is highly treatable.

2. First Phase:

The tumor is localized to the skin and is smaller than a certain thickness.

Excellent prognosis with a high likelihood of recovery. Overall, there is a high observed 5-year survival rate.

3. Stage Two:

The tumor's features include thickness, ulceration, and potential lymph node dissemination.

Prognosis: Treatment options include surgically removing the main tumor and, if required, dissecting lymph nodes. Compared to Stage I, the 5-year survival rate is somewhat lower.

4. Stage Three:

The cancer has either spread to nearby lymph nodes or formed satellite lesions.

Prognosis: The 5-year survival rate is lower than in the early periods. Treatment options include adjuvant medications, surgery, and lymph node dissection.

5. Phase Four:

The cancer has spread to distant organs or lymph nodes that were not near the original tumor.

Prognosis: In general, the prognosis is less good and the 5-year survival rate is lower. Treatment options may include systemic medicines including immunotherapy, targeted therapy, chemotherapy, and other techniques.

6. Metastatic melanoma:

Description: The cancer returned after the initial course of treatment.

The location and severity of the recurrence will determine the prognosis. There are numerous options for treatment, such as systemic medicines, radiation, and surgery.

Elements of Prediction:

Tumor Thickness: Thicker tumors typically have worse prognoses.

Ulceration: If there is ulceration, or the skin breakdown above the tumor, the prognosis is worse.

Mitotic Rate: The rate at which tumor cells divide can affect the prognosis.

Lymph Node Involvement: The presence of cancer cells in the surrounding lymph nodes is a significant factor.

Metastasis: The cancer's capacity to spread to distant organs has a significant influence on the prognosis.

It's important to keep in mind that personal factors like age, overall health, and treatment response can have an impact on prognosis. Better outcomes for melanoma patients depend on early detection and treatment. Regular surveillance and follow-up are often recommended, especially for individuals with a history of melanoma.

Treatment Options

Treatment for melanoma depends on several factors, including the patient's overall health, the location of the tumor, and the cancer's stage. Treatment options may include a combination of targeted medicines, systemic therapy, and surgery. Some common treatment options for melanoma include the following:

CHAPTER THREE

1. Surgery:

Wide Local Excision: The primary tumor and a margin of healthy tissue are surgically excised in order to ensure complete removal.

Sentinel Lymph Node Biopsy: The lymph node or nodes closest to the primary tumor are removed and analyzed in order to determine whether the cancer has spread.

2. Immunotherapy:

Checkpoint inhibitors: Drugs such as pembrolizumab and nivolumab block specific proteins (PD-1 or PD-L1) to enhance the immune system's ability to recognize and destroy cancer cells.

Interleukin-2 (IL-2): High-dose interleukin-2 therapy can cause the immune system to target melanoma cells.

3. Personalized Health Care:

BRAF Inhibitors: Drugs like vemurafenib and dabrafenib work by targeting the particular genetic mutation (BRAF mutation) that causes melanoma, so preventing the cancer from spreading.

MEK Inhibitors: In addition to BRAF inhibitors, medications like as trametinib may be utilized to further target specific pathways associated with the development of melanoma.

4. Chemotherapy:

Systemic Chemotherapy: Although it is sometimes used, conventional chemotherapy is mostly reserved for cases of melanoma that have progressed.

5. Radiation Therapy:

Adjuvant Radiation: In order to target any remaining cancer cells or lymph nodes, radiation therapy may be used after surgery.

Advanced cancers can be treated with palliative radiation treatment to lessen symptoms and limit their spread.

6. Clinical Assessments:

Research Protocols: Enrolling in clinical trials gives access to novel therapies and advances the field of melanoma research.

7. Treatment for Adversive Melanoma:

Combination Therapies: Some patients with advanced melanoma may get both targeted treatment and immunotherapy.

Second-Line Therapies: If the cancer reappears or if the initial therapies fail, medical specialists may investigate other options for treatment.

8. Healthcare Assistance:

Palliative care offers supportive treatment and symptom relief with the goal of enhancing the quality of life for individuals with advanced melanoma.

Psychosocial support: Emotional and psychological support must be a part of the whole care plan.

9. Treatment-free remission (TFR):

Observation Periods: Some patients may experience an observation time after a successful course of therapy, during which they are not given any medicine. We call this remission that doesn't require treatment.

The distinct features of the melanoma, such as its stage, location, and genetic composition, determine the best course of treatment. The choices for treatments are highly personalized. In interdisciplinary teams, dermatologists, surgeons, medical oncologists, and other experts create customized treatment plans for melanoma patients. The key to improving outcomes is early discovery and quick response.

Avoidance and Sunscreen Use

Reducing your chance of developing this type of skin cancer primarily involves avoiding melanoma and using sunscreen sparingly. The following are crucial safety measures and recommendations for the sun:

1. Application of Sunscreen:

Broad-Spectrum Protection: Use a broad-spectrum sunscreen with an SPF (Sun Protection Factor) of at least thirty to protect yourself from UVA and UVB rays.

Usage Guidelines: Apply generously and reapply sunscreen every two hours, or more frequently if you swim or perspire.

2. Donning protective attire:

Wear Hats: Wide-brimmed hats provide protection for the face, neck, and ears.

Long Sleeves and Pants: Wear lightweight long sleeves and pants to minimize your exposure to the sun.

3. Seek out shade.

Avoid the Highest Sun Hours: Find cover, especially from 10 a.m. and 3 p.m. and 4:00 p.m.

Use Sunshades and Umbrellas: When you're outside, search for shade from sunshades and umbrellas.

4. Sunglasses:

UV-Blocking Sunglasses: Use sunglasses that block UVA and UVB rays to protect your eyes and the skin around them.

5. Restrict the Use of Sunbeds:

Avoid tanning beds: they are associated with an increased risk of skin cancer and produce harmful UV radiation.

6. Regular Skin Examinations:

Self-Examinations: Regularly examine your skin to look for moles and any changes in its appearance.

Expert Skin Examinations: Schedule a regular skin examination with a dermatologist, especially if there are additional risk factors or a family history of melanoma.

7. Retain Hydration:

Hydrate Your Skin: Drink plenty of water to keep your skin moisturized and to promote overall skin health.

8. Discover for Yourself:

Learn the ABCDE Rule: To diagnose melanoma, one must be aware of the ABCDE rule, which includes Asymmetry, Border irregularity, Color variations, Diameter more than a pencil eraser, and Evolution or changes over time.

9. Avoid getting sunburned:

Avoiding sunburns is crucial since they increase the risk of developing melanoma.

10. Regular exams of the eyes:

Eye Protection: To protect your eyes from UV rays, wear sunglasses.

It is important to schedule routine eye exams, especially if there are concerns regarding vision changes or the condition of your eyes.

11. Knowledge of the Community:

Encourage Sun Safety: Raise awareness of the risks associated with extended sun exposure and advocate for laws in your community that support sun safety.

12. Adhere to the Guidelines for Children:

Children's Sun Protection: Especially during the hottest hours of the day, protect children from the sun by using sunscreen, covering themselves with protective clothes, and avoiding exposing them to it.

13. Acknowledge Your Danger:

Identify Risk Factors: Be aware of the risks associated with your own skin tone, fair complexion, and a family history of sunburns.

By including these sun protection measures into your daily routine and keeping an eye out for any changes in your skin, you may reduce your risk of melanoma and enhance the general health of your skin. Regular sun safety measures not only prevent melanoma but also lower the risk of other skin cancers and improve long-term health.

Handling Melanoma

After a melanoma diagnosis, it's critical to address the practical, psychological, and physical aspects of the trip. Here are a few coping strategies for melanoma:

1. Obtain Psychological Support:

Talk to Loved Ones: Share your thoughts and feelings with your friends and relatives.

Join assistance Groups: To share experiences and get assistance, connect with other melanoma survivors.

Therapy or Counseling: Consider obtaining professional counseling or therapy to assist in coping with the emotional impact of the diagnosis.

2. Discover for Yourself:

Acknowledge the Diagnosis: Become knowledgeable about melanoma, its treatments, and what to expect while driving.

Ask Questions: Please don't hesitate to ask your medical team any questions you may have about your diagnosis, prognosis, and available treatments.

3. Keep up the Open Communication:

Communication with Healthcare Team: Make sure you and your team of physicians and nurses are in continual communication. Discuss any concerns, negative effects, or changes to your health.

4. Set logical goals:

Take It One Step at a Time: Break up challenging tasks and issues into smaller, more manageable steps.

appreciate successes: Express gratitude and appreciate small obstacles encountered along the way.

5. Give Yourself First Aid:

Physical Well-Being: Take good care of your body by eating a balanced diet, exercising frequently, and drinking lots of water (as recommended by your healthcare team).

Rest and Sleep: Make sure you give yourself enough time and attention to get enough sleep.

6. Analyze Mind-Body Techniques:

Practice mindfulness or meditation to lower stress and improve mental health.

Engage in yoga or mild exercise: Engage in activities that promote relaxation and increased flexibility.

7. Maintain a Robust Support System:

Stay in Touch with Others: Continue your bonds with family members who are sympathetic and understanding.

Helpful Professionals: Seek guidance from a social worker, therapist, or counselor who specializes in cancer treatment.

8. Managing Your Fear and Anxiety:

Managing Fear and Anxiety: Acknowledge and address any concerns you may have regarding the diagnosis. Consider techniques such as visualization and deep breathing.

9. Examine Your Creative Sources:

Try your hand at writing, music, or art as a means of expressing yourself and letting go of your feelings.

CHAPTER FOUR

10. Stay Up to Date on Treatment Information:

Being Aware of Your therapy: Stay informed on the course of your therapy, any potential side effects, and what to anticipate moving forward.

11. Create a Future Strategy:

Establish Future Goals: Plan for the future and set realistic goals for yourself.

Survivorship Planning: Work with your medical team to create a plan for post-treatment care and monitoring.

12. Advocate for Yourself:

Active Involvement: Be proactive in selecting the course of your medical care and treatment.

Seek Second Opinions: If required, seek second opinions to ensure that the decisions you are making are well-informed.

13. Pay tribute to important anniversaries:

Milestone Recognition: Acknowledge and celebrate any milestone, whether it has to do with treatment, recovery, or personal achievement.

14. Analyze Religious Traditions:

Spiritual Well-Being: Engage in activities that align with your spiritual beliefs for further assistance.

Fulfilling both physical and emotional needs is a journey in managing melanoma. Being informed, prioritizing self-care, and maintaining a strong support system can all help one become more resilient and in charge of how they manage the challenges posed by melanoma.

Aftercare and Resilience in Treatment

Following a melanoma diagnosis, survivability and follow-up care are important aspects of the process. Important elements for survivorship and after-treatment care are as follows:

1. Regular Follow-Up Sessions:

Visits with Dermatologists and Oncologists: Maintain regular follow-up appointments with your dermatologist and oncologist to monitor any changes in your skin or signs of a recurrence.

Frequency of Visits: The number of follow-up visits may vary depending on an individual's characteristics and the stage of the melanoma.

2. Imaging and Check-Ups:

Imaging tests: Imaging tests such as CT, PET, or MRI scans may occasionally be carried out to look for any signs of metastasis.

Blood Tests: Regular blood tests may be recommended to check for any irregularities.

3. Skin Self-Examinations:

Regular Self-Examinations: Continue to examine your skin frequently to detect any changes, newly formed moles, or dubious lesions.

Educate Yourself: Stay informed on the ABCDE rule for melanoma detection and report any concerning changes to your healthcare provider.

4. Sun Protection:

Year-Round Sun Safety: To reduce your risk of getting new skin cancers, protect yourself from the sun by wearing protective clothing, applying sunscreen, and seeking out shade.

Avoid Tanning Beds: Using tanning beds increases your chance of getting skin cancer.

5. Emotional and Psychological Wellbeing:

Supportive Resources: To receive emotional and psychological support, continue attending support groups, counseling, or therapy.

Managing Anxiety and Fear: Manage any anxiety or fear related to the cancer journey. Experts in support services can assist in overcoming survivor-related challenges.

6. Selecting a Healthier Way of Living:

Balanced Diet: Maintain a healthy, well-balanced diet to enhance overall wellbeing.

Regular Exercise: Follow your doctor's advice and engage in regular exercise to maintain your physical health.

7. Education and Advocacy:

Keep Up: Stay informed about melanoma, issues surrounding survivability, and any developments in treatment or research.

Advocacy: You could decide to focus on preventing and increasing awareness of skin cancer.

8. Getting along with the medical personnel:

Maintain Open Lines of Communication: Inform your healthcare staff of any symptoms, concerns, or changes in your health.

Share Your Concerns: If you have any particular worries regarding survivorship or if your therapy is causing you any negative effects, please let your healthcare practitioners know.

9. Watch out for any aftereffects:

Late Effects of Treatment: Be aware of any potential pharmaceutical side effects, and immediately let your healthcare provider know if you experience any new symptoms.

10. bolstering connections

Keep in Touch with Other Survivors: Stay in touch with other melanoma survivors to share experiences and lend support to each other.

Community Resources: Seek out nearby resources that provide cancer survivors with assistance.

11. Analyzing Possible Secondary Cancers

Screening for Other malignancies: Depending on the patient's risk factors and the specific cancer treatment they have received, it may be recommended to screen for additional malignancies.

12. Strategies for Afterlife Care:

Tailored Plans: Work with your medical team to develop a survivorship care plan that outlines necessary medical attention, potential risks, and lifestyle advice.

Managing the practical, emotional, and physical facets of life is a unique and ongoing process that follows cancer treatment. A more empowered and healthier survivorship experience is the result of self-monitoring, regular follow-up therapy, and a proactive approach to overall well-being.

CONCLUSION

In conclusion, melanoma is a serious form of skin cancer that necessitates comprehensive understanding, early detection, and a multidisciplinary approach to treatment. Navigating the path of melanoma involves many considerations, from diagnosis to treatment and survivorship.

Key takeaways:

Early Diagnosis is Critical: Melanoma is more curable when detected early, which is why self-examinations on a regular basis and adherence to the ABCDE rule are crucial.

Staging Affects Prognosis: Based on the characteristics and location of the tumor, staging affects treatment options.

Treatment Options Are Various: Immunotherapy, targeted therapy, surgical excision, lymph node biopsies, and, in some cases, chemotherapy or radiation are some of the options available.

Sun Safety Is Preventive: Adopt sun safety practices like applying sunscreen, donning protective clothing, and avoiding tanning salons to reduce your chance of developing melanoma.

Suffering and Triumph are Personal Journeys: Coping with a melanoma diagnosis necessitates informational support, emotional support, and self-care. Survivorship requires regular follow-up care, ongoing monitoring, and a focus on overall wellness.

Throughout the process, it is imperative to have support networks, maintain open communication with medical personnel, and take an active role in one's own care. People who are better educated are better able to advocate for themselves, make informed decisions, and actively participate in their treatment plans.

Research is continuing to change the state of melanoma treatment, offering hope for improved survivability and prognoses. Each person's experience with melanoma is unique, but with early detection, comprehensive care, and a wholistic approach to health, individuals can

surmount challenges and pursue a high quality of
life even after being diagnosed.

THE END